The Ultimate Lean & Green Main & Side Dish Cookbook

Easy Lean & Green Main & Side Dish Recipes For Beginners

Jesse Cohen

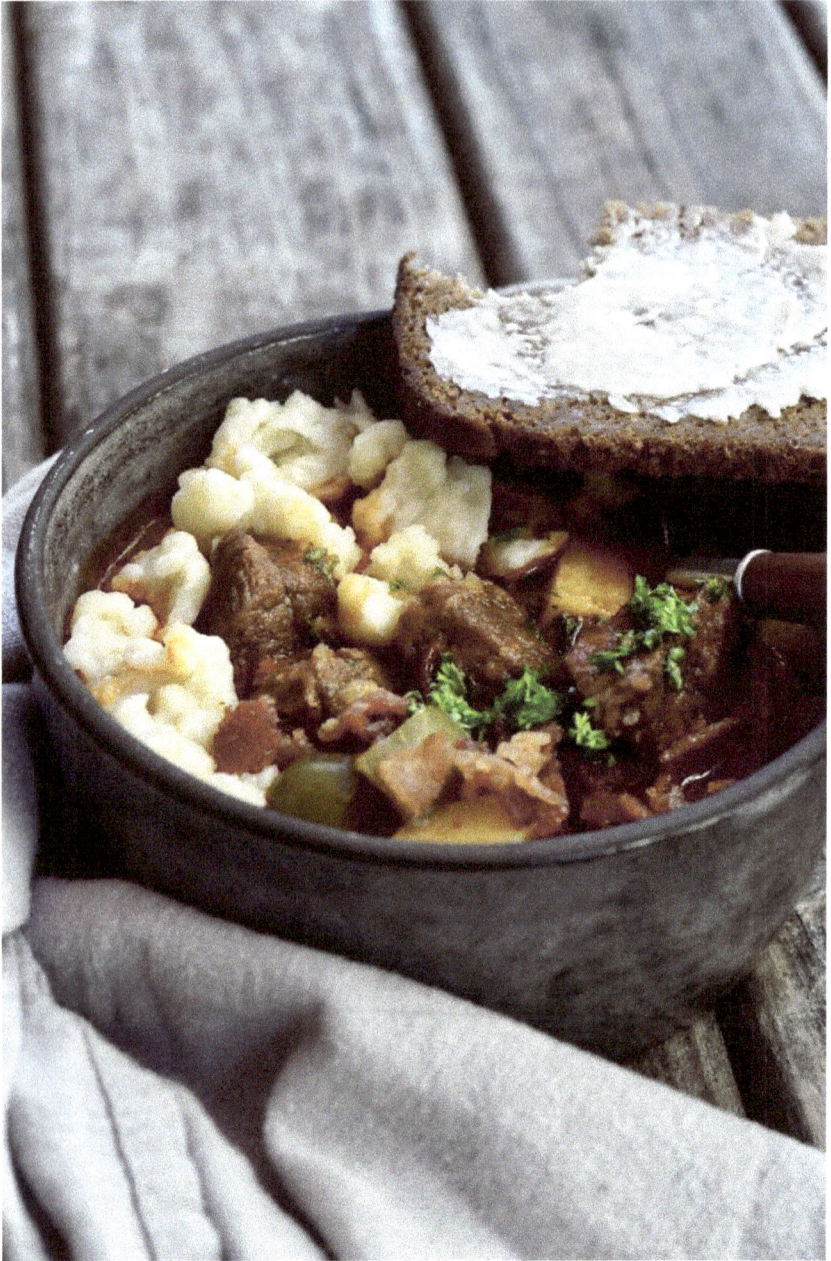

Table of contents

Brooke's Chili

Preparation Time:

Cooking Time: 1 hour

Servings: 4

Ingredients:

- 2 lb. of organic ground beef
- 1 diced onion
- 3 cloves of minced garlic
- 6 diced tomatoes
- 1 jar of tomato sauce
- 1 tablespoon of salt
- 1 cup of water
- 1 cup of kidney beans soaked in water overnight (drained)
- 1 cup of pinto beans soaked in water overnight (drained)
- 2 tablespoons of chili powder
- 1 tablespoon of cumin
- 1 tablespoon of honey or maple syrup
- 1 teaspoon of baking stevia

- 1 teaspoon of pepper

Directions:

1. In a large pot, brown the ground beef and drain the oil.
2. Add the onion and garlic and cook until translucent.
3. Add the rest of the ingredients and simmer for 1 hour.

Nutrition:

- Calories: 110
- Fat: 31 g
- Fiber: 18 g
- Carbs: 15 g
- Protein: 12 g

Flavorful Broccoli Soup

Preparation Time: 10 minutes

Cooking Time: 4 hours 15 minutes

Servings: 6

Ingredients:

- 20 oz. of broccoli florets

- 4 oz. of cream cheese

- 8 oz. of cheddar cheese; shredded

- 1/2 tsp. of paprika

- 1/2 tsp. of ground mustard

- 3 cups of chicken stock

- 2 garlic cloves; chopped

- 1 onion; diced

- 1 cup of carrots; shredded

- 1/4 tsp. of baking soda

- 1/4 tsp. of salt

Directions:

1. Add all the ingredients except cream cheese and cheddar cheese to a Crock Pot and stir well.
2. Cover and cook on low for 4 hours.
3. Purée the soup using an immersion blender until it's smooth.
4. Stir in the cream cheese and cheddar cheese.
5. Cover and cook on low for 15 minutes more.
6. Season with pepper and salt.
7. Serve and enjoy.

Nutrition:

- Calories 275
- Fat 19 g
- Carbohydrates 19 g
- Sugar 4 g
- Protein 14 g
- Cholesterol 60 mg

Lentil Soup

Preparation Time:

Cooking Time: 2 hours

Servings: 4

Ingredients:

- 2 tablespoons of olive oil
- 2 chopped onions
- 1 chopped red pepper
- 1 chopped carrot
- 2 cloves of minced garlic
- ½ teaspoon of cumin
- ¾ teaspoon of thyme
- 1 bay leaf
- 8 cups of chicken broth
- 2 chopped tomatoes
- ½ pound of dried lentils (1¼ cup)
- Optional: add bacon or ham to flavor.
- 1 teaspoon of salt

- ¼ teaspoon of pepper
- Handful of spinach

Directions:

1. Sauté vegetables in oil.
2. Mix all the ingredients (except spinach and spices).
3. Cover and cook on low for 2 hours.
4. Add spinach and spices.

Nutrition:

- Calories: 257
- Fat: 13 g
- Fiber: 37 g
- Carbs: 11g
- Protein: 8 g

White Chicken Chili

Preparation Time:

Cooking Time: 30 minutes

Servings: 4

Ingredients:

- 1 tablespoon of olive oil
- 1 pound of chicken strips cut into pieces
- 2 teaspoons of cumin
- ½ teaspoon of oregano
- ½ teaspoon of salt
- ½ teaspoon of pepper
- 1 chopped onion
- 1 chopped red bell pepper
- 4 cloves of minced garlic
- 4 cups of chicken broth
- 2 cups of northern beans soaked in water overnight (drained)

Directions:

1. Sauté chicken and spices in oil and remove from pan.
2. Sauté onion and red pepper.
3. Add all of the ingredients including chicken into a pot and cook on medium-low heat for 15 minutes.

Nutrition:

- Calories: 208
- Fat: 3 g
- Fiber: 4 g
- Carbs: 7 g
- Protein: 27 g

Black Bean Soup

Preparation Time: 5 minutes

Cooking Time: 1 hour

Servings: 4

Ingredients:

- 1 pound of dry black beans (soak in water overnight and drain water)
- 1 tablespoon of olive oil
- 2 cups of chopped onion or 1 leek
- 1 cup of chopped carrots
- 4 cloves of minced garlic
- 2 teaspoons of cumin
- ¼ teaspoon of red pepper flakes
- 4 cups of chicken broth
- 4 cups of water
- ¼ teaspoon of thyme
- 2 chopped tomatoes or 1 (14 oz.) can tomatoes
- 1½ teaspoon of salt

- Optional: add bacon or ham to flavor.
- Chopped green onions to garnish

Directions:

Sauté vegetables in oil. Add all of the ingredients and cook on stovetop on medium-low heat for 1 hour.

Nutrition:

- Calories: 508
- Fat: 12 g
- Fiber: 9 g
- Carbs: 24 g
- Protein: 40 g

Homemade Vegetable Broth

Preparation Time: 5 minutes

Cooking Time: 30 minutes

Servings: 4

Ingredients:

- 1 tablespoon of olive oil

- 1 chopped onion

- 2 chopped stalks celery

- 2 chopped carrots

- 1 head of bok choy

- 6 cups or 1 package fresh spinach

- 2+ quarts of water

- 1 tablespoon of salt

- ½ teaspoon of pepper

- 1 teaspoon fresh sage

Directions:

1. Sauté vegetables in oil. Add water and simmer for 1 hour.

2. Keep adding water as required.
3. Pour broth mixture into pint and quart mason jars.
4. Leave one full inch of space from the top of the jar or it will crack when it freezes and liquid expand. Jars can stay in freezer for up to a year.
5. Take out and use whenever you make a soup.

Nutrition:

- Calories: 140
- Fat: 2 g
- Fiber: 23 g
- Carbs: 22 g
- Protein: 47 g

Tasty Basil Tomato Soup

Preparation Time: 10 minutes

Cooking Time: 6 hours

Servings: 6

Ingredients:

- 28 oz. of can whole peeled tomatoes
- 1/2 cup of fresh basil leaves
- 4 cups of chicken stock
- 1 tsp. of red pepper flakes
- 3 garlic cloves; peeled
- 2 onions; diced
- 3 carrots; peeled and diced
- 3 tbsps. of olive oil
- 1 tsp. of salt

Directions:

1. Add all ingredients to a Crock Pot and stir well.
2. Cover and cook on low for 6 hours.

3. Purée the soup until smooth using an immersion blender.

4. Season soup with pepper and salt.

5. Serve and enjoy.

Nutrition:

- Calories 126
- Fat 5 g
- Carbohydrates 13 g
- Sugar 7 g
- Protein 5 g
- Cholesterol 0 mg

Mixed Vegetable Soup

Preparation Time: 5 minutes

Cooking Time: 30 minutes

Servings: 4

Ingredients:

- 1 tablespoon of olive oil
- 1 chopped leek
- 1 chopped bok choy
- 4 chopped carrots
- 2 cloves of minced garlic
- 1 chopped zucchini
- 2 chopped tomatoes
- 1 cup of garbanzo beans soaked in water overnight (drained)
- 5 chopped potatoes
- 8 cups of broth
- 1 teaspoon of basil
- ½ cup of amaranth

Directions:

1. Sauté the first four ingredients, adding garlic in the last minute.
2. Add the rest of the ingredients and simmer on the stove for 25 minutes.

Nutrition:

- Calories: 241
- Fat: 2 g
- Fiber: 16 g
- Carbs: 9 g
- Protein: 22 g

Coconut and Shrimp Bisque

Preparation Time: 10 minutes

Cooking Time: 15 minutes

Servings: 4

Ingredients:

- ¼ cup of red curry paste
- 2 tablespoons of water
- 1 tablespoon of extra-virgin olive oil
- 1 bunch of scallions; sliced
- 1-pound medium (21-30 count) of shrimp; peeled and deveined
- 1 cup of frozen peas
- 1 red bell pepper; diced
- 1 (14-ounce) can of full-fat coconut milk
- Kosher salt

Directions:

1. In a small bowl, whisk together the red curry paste and water. Set aside.

2. Select roast/sauté and set to med. Press start/stop to start. Allow to preheat for 3 minutes.
3. Add the oil and scallions. Cook for 2 minutes.
4. Add the shrimp, peas, and bell pepper. Stir well to mix. Stir in the red curry paste. Cook for 5 minutes, or until the peas are soft.
5. Stir in coconut milk and cook for more 5 minutes or until shrimp is cooked through and the bisque is thoroughly heated.
6. Season with salt and serve immediately.

Nutrition:

- Calories: 460
- Total Fat: 32 g
- Saturated Fat: 23 g
- Cholesterol: 223 mg
- Sodium: 902 mg
- Carbohydrates: 16 g
- Fiber: 5 g
- Protein: 29 g

Healthy Chicken Kale Soup

Preparation Time: 10 minutes

Cooking Time: 6 hours 15 minutes

Servings: 6

Ingredients:

- 2 lb. of chicken breasts; skinless and boneless
- 1/4 cup of fresh lemon juice
- 5 oz. of baby kale
- 32 oz. of chicken stock
- 1/2 cup of olive oil
- 1 large onion; sliced
- 14 oz. of chicken broth
- 1 tbsp. of extra-virgin olive oil
- Salt

Directions:

1. Heat the extra-virgin olive oil in a pan over medium heat.
2. Season chicken with salt and place in the hot pan.
3. Cover pan and cook chicken for 15 minutes.

4. Remove chicken from the pan and shred it using forks.
5. Add shredded chicken to a Crock Pot.
6. Add sliced onion, olive oil, and broth to a blender and blend until properly mixed.
7. Pour blended mixture into the Crock Pot.
8. Add the remaining ingredients to the Crock Pot and stir well.
9. Cover and cook on low for 6 hours.
10. Stir well and serve.

Nutrition:

- Calories 493
- Fat 33 g
- Carbohydrates 8 g
- Sugar 9 g
- Protein 47 g
- Cholesterol 135 mg

Potato Soup

Preparation Time: 5 minutes

Cooking Time: 30 minutes

Servings: 4

Ingredients:

- 2 tablespoons of olive oil
- 1 diced onion
- 4 minced cloves of garlic
- 1 teaspoon of thyme
- 1 bay leaf
- 4 diced red potatoes
- 6 cups of water
- 1 sliced leek
- 3 diced celery stalks
- 2 teaspoons of salt
- ¼ teaspoon of pepper

Directions:

1. Sauté onion, garlic, thyme, and bay leaf in oil until translucent.
2. Add the rest of the ingredients and simmer for about 20 minutes.

Nutrition:

- Calories: 267
- Fat: 13 g
- Fiber: 14 g
- Carbs: 17 g
- Protein: 10 g

Richard's Best Chicken

Preparation Time: 5 minutes

Cooking Time: 30 minutes

Servings: 4

Ingredients:

- 2 tablespoons of olive oil
- 8 chicken thighs
- 6 cloves of garlic
- 1 jar of artichoke hearts; drained
- ¾ cup of chicken broth
- 3 fresh squeezed oranges
- 1 sliced Meyer lemon
- ¼ cup of capers
- ½ cup of lives

Directions:

1. In a cast-iron skillet, fry chicken on all sides in oil until skin is golden and crispy. Remove from skillet.

2. Sauté garlic and artichokes for a couple of minutes, add chicken (skin up). Pour in the rest of the ingredients and bring to a boil.
3. Place skillet with all ingredients uncovered in a 350° F oven for 30 minutes.

Nutrition:

- Calories: 285
- Fat: 28 g
- Fiber: 7 g
- Carbs: 34 g
- Protein: 23 g

Lamb Stew

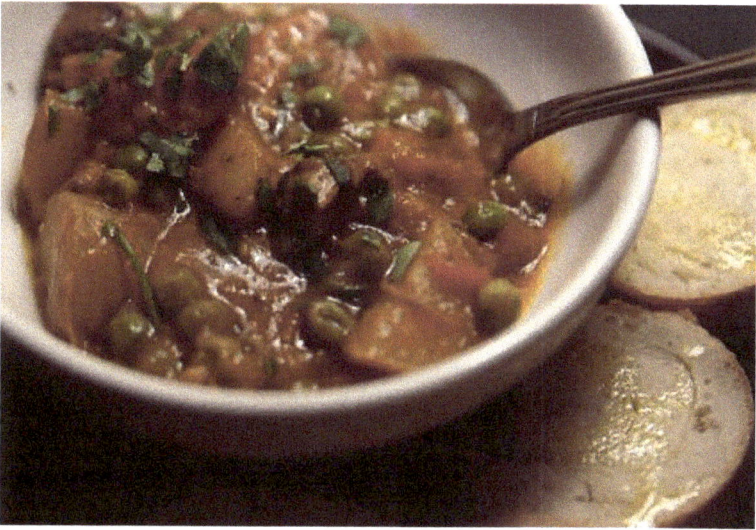

Preparation Time: 10 minutes

Cooking Time: 8 hours

Servings: 2

Ingredients:

- 1/2 lb. of lean lamb; boneless and cubed

- 2 tbsps. of lemon juice

- 1/2 onion; chopped

- 2 garlic cloves; minced

- 2 fresh thyme sprigs
- 1/4 tsp. of turmeric
- 1/4 cup of green olives; sliced
- 1/2 tsp. of black pepper
- 1/4 tsp. of salt

Directions:

1. Add all the ingredients into a crock pot and stir well.
2. Cover and cook on low for 8 hours.
3. Stir well and serve.

Nutrition:

- Calories 297
- Fat 20.3 g
- Carbohydrates 4 g
- Sugar 5 g
- Protein 21 g
- Cholesterol 80 mg

Goulash

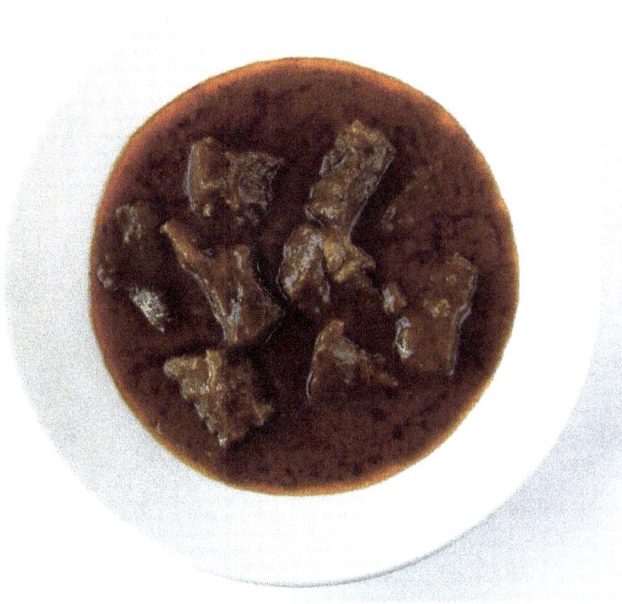

Preparation Time: 15 minutes

Cooking Time: 55 minutes

Servings: 6

Ingredients:

- ½ cup all-purpose flour
- 1 tablespoon of kosher salt
- ½ teaspoon of freshly ground black pepper

- 2 pounds of beef stew meat

- 2 tablespoons of canola oil

- 1 medium red bell pepper; seeded and chopped

- 4 garlic cloves; minced

- 1 large yellow onion; diced

- 2 tablespoons of smoked paprika

- 1½ pounds of small Yukon gold potatoes; halved

- 2 cups of beef broth

- 2 tablespoons of tomato paste

- ¼ cup of sour cream Fresh parsley, for garnish

Directions:

1. Select burn/sauté and set to start. Press start/stop to start. Allow to preheat for 5 minutes.
2. Mix together the flour, salt, and pepper in a small bowl. Dip the pieces of beef into the flour mixture, shaking off any extra flour.
3. Add the oil and allow to heat for 1 minute. Place the meat in the pot and brown it on all sides, for about 10 minutes.
4. Add the bell pepper, garlic, onion, and smoked paprika. Sauté for about 8 minutes or until the onion is translucent.
5. Add the potatoes, beef stock, and ingredient and stir.

6. Select pressure and set to low. Set time to 30 minutes. Select start/stop to start.

7. When the pressure cooking is finished, relieve the pressure by moving the pressure discharge valve to the vent position. Cautiously remove top unit where heat passes through while delivering pressure.

8. Add the soured cream and blend thoroughly. Garnish with parsley, if desired, and serve immediately.

Nutrition:

- Calories: 413
- Fat: 13 g
- Saturated fat: 4 g
- Cholesterol: 98 mg
- Sodium: 432 mg
- Carbohydrates: 64 g
- Fiber: 5 g
- Protein: 37 g

Loaded Potato Soup

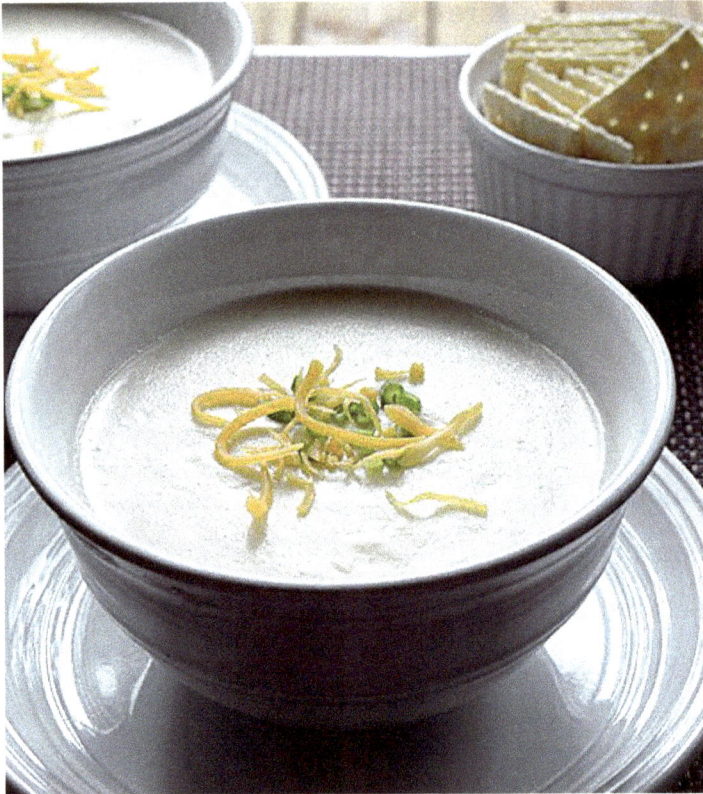

Preparation Time: 15 minutes

Cooking Time: 30 minutes

Servings: 6

Ingredients:

- 5 slices of bacon; chopped

- 1 onion; chopped

- 3 garlic cloves; minced

- 4 pounds of russet potatoes; peeled and chopped

- 4 cups of chicken broth

- 1 cup of whole milk

- ½ teaspoon of sea salt

- ½ teaspoon of freshly ground black pepper

- 1½ cups of shredded cheddar cheese

- Sour cream; for serving (optional)

- Chopped fresh chives; for serving (optional)

Directions:

1. Add the bacon, onion, and garlic. Cook for 5 minutes, stirring occasionally. Put aside some of the bacon for garnish.
2. Add the potatoes and chicken stock. Setup pressure lid, making sure the pressure release valve is in the seal position.
3. Select pressure and set to high. Set time to 10 minutes, then press start/stop to start.
4. At the point when pressure cooking is finished, fast relieve the pressure by moving the pressure discharge valve to the

vent position. Cautiously remove top unit where heat passes through while delivering pressure.

5. Add the milk and mash the ingredients until the soup reaches your required consistency. Season with the salt and black pepper. Sprinkle the cheese evenly over the top of the soup. Close crisping lid.

6. Select broil and set time to 5 minutes. Press start/stop to start.

7. When cooking is complete, top with the reserved crispy bacon and serve with soured cream and chives (if using).

Nutrition:

- Calories: 468
- Total fat: 19 g
- Saturated fat: 9 g
- Cholesterol: 51 mg
- Sodium: 1041 mg
- Carbohydrates: 53 g
- Fiber: 8 g
- Protein: 23 g

Butternut Squash, Apple, Bacon and Orzo Soup

Preparation Time: 10 minutes

Cooking Time: 28 minutes

Servings: 8

Ingredients:

- 4 slices of uncooked bacon; cut into ½-inch pieces
- 12 ounces of butternut squash; peeled and cubed
- 1 green apple; cut into small cubes
- Kosher salt
- Freshly ground black pepper
- 1 tablespoon of minced fresh oregano
- 2 quarts (64 ounces) of chicken stock
- 1 cup of orzo

Directions:

1. Select roast/sauté and set temperature to high. Press start/stop to start. Allow to preheat for 5 minutes.

2. Place the bacon in the pot and cook, stirring frequently, for about 5 minutes, or until fat is produced and the bacon starts to brown. Using a slotted spoon, transfer the bacon to a paper towel-lined plate to drain, leaving the rendered bacon fat in the pot.

3. Add the butternut squash, apple, salt, pepper, and sauté until partially soft, or for about 5 minutes. Stir in the oregano.

4. Add the bacon back to the pot alongside the chicken broth. Bring to a boil for about 10 minutes, then add the orzo. Cook for about 8 minutes, or until the orzo is soft. Serve.

Nutrition:

- Calories: 247
- Total Fat: 7 g
- Saturated Fat: 2 g
- Cholesterol: 17 mg
- Sodium: 563 mg
- Carbohydrates: 33 g
- Fiber: 3 g
- Protein: 12 g

Delicious Chicken Soup

Preparation Time: 10 minutes

Cooking Time: 4 hours 30 minutes

Servings: 4

Ingredients:

- 1 lb. of chicken breasts; boneless and skinless
- 2 tbsp. of fresh basil; chopped
- 1 1/2 cups of mozzarella cheese; shredded
- 2 garlic cloves; minced
- 1 tbsp. of Parmesan cheese; grated
- 2 tbsp. of dried basil
- 2 cups of chicken stock
- 28 oz. of tomatoes; diced
- 1/4 tsp. of pepper
- 1/2 tsp. of salt

Directions:

1. Add chicken, Parmesan cheese, dried basil, tomatoes, garlic, pepper, and salt to a Crock Pot and stir well to mix.
2. Cover and cook on low for 4 hours.
3. Add fresh basil and mozzarella cheese and stir well.
4. Cover again and cook for 30 more minutes or until cheese is melted.
5. Remove chicken from the Crock Pot and shred using fork.
6. Return shredded chicken to the Crock Pot and stir to mix.
7. Serve and enjoy.

Nutrition:

- Calories: 299
- Fat: 16 g
- Carbohydrates: 3 g
- Sugar: 6 g
- Protein: 38 g
- Cholesterol: 108 mg

Spicy Chicken Pepper Stew

Preparation Time: 10 minutes

Cooking Time: 6 hours

Servings: 6

Ingredients:

- 3 chicken breasts; skinless and boneless, cut into small pieces
- 1 tsp. of garlic; minced
- 1 tsp. of ground ginger
- 2 tsp. of olive oil
- 2 tsp. of soy sauce
- 1 tbsp. of fresh lemon juice
- 1/2 cup of green onions; sliced
- 1 tbsp. of crushed red pepper
- 8 oz. of chicken stock
- 1 bell pepper; chopped
- 1 green chili pepper; sliced
- 2 jalapeño peppers; sliced

- 1/2 tsp. of black pepper

- 1/4 tsp. of sea salt

Directions:

1. Add all ingredients to a large bowl and blend well. Place in the refrigerator overnight.
2. Pour marinated chicken mixture into a Crock Pot.
3. Cover and cook on low for 6 hours.
4. Stir well and serve.

Nutrition:

- Calories: 171
- Fat: 4 g
- Carbohydrates: 7 g
- Sugar: 7 g
- Protein: 22 g
- Cholesterol: 65 mg

Beef Chili

Preparation Time: 10 minutes

Cooking Time: 8 hours

Servings: 6

Ingredients:

- 1 lb. of ground beef
- 1 tsp. of garlic powder
- 1 tsp. of paprika
- 3 tsp. of chili powder
- 1 tbsp. of Worcestershire sauce
- 1 tbsp. of fresh parsley; chopped
- 1 tsp. of onion powder
- 25 oz. of tomatoes; chopped
- 4 carrots; chopped
- 1 onion; diced
- 1 bell pepper; diced
- 1/2 tsp. of sea salt

Directions:

1. Brown the ground meat in a pan over high heat until meat is no longer pink.
2. Transfer meat to a Crock Pot.
3. Add bell pepper, tomatoes, carrots, and onion to the Crock Pot and stir well.
4. Add the remaining ingredients and stir well.
5. Cover and cook on low for 8 hours.
6. Serve and enjoy.

Nutrition:

- Calories: 152
- Fat: 4 g
- Carbohydrates: 4 g
- Sugar: 8 g
- Protein: 18 g
- Cholesterol 51 mg

Healthy Spinach Soup

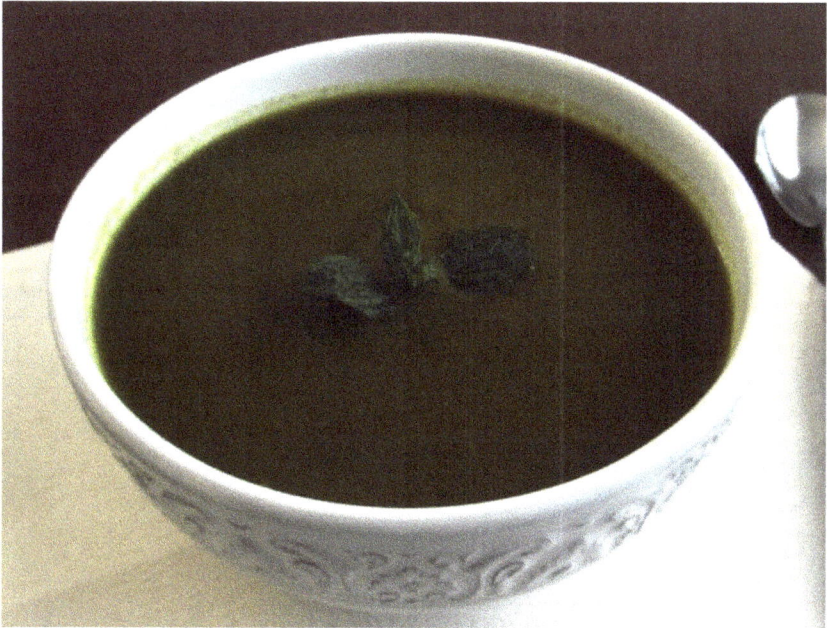

Preparation Time: 10 minutes

Cooking Time: 3 hours

Servings: 8

Ingredients:

- 3 cups of frozen spinach; chopped, thawed, and drained

- 8 oz. of cheddar cheese; shredded

- 1 egg; lightly beaten

- 10 oz. of can cream chicken soup
- 8 oz. of cream cheese; softened

Directions:

1. Add spinach to a large bowl. Purée the spinach.
2. Add egg, chicken soup, cheese, and pepper to the spinach purée and blend well.
3. Transfer spinach mixture to a Crock Pot.
4. Cover and cook on low for 3 hours.
5. Stir in cheddar and serve.

Nutrition:

- Calories: 256
- Fat: 29 g
- Carbohydrates: 1 g
- Sugar: 0.5 g
- Protein: 11 g
- Cholesterol: 84 mg

Mexican Chicken Soup

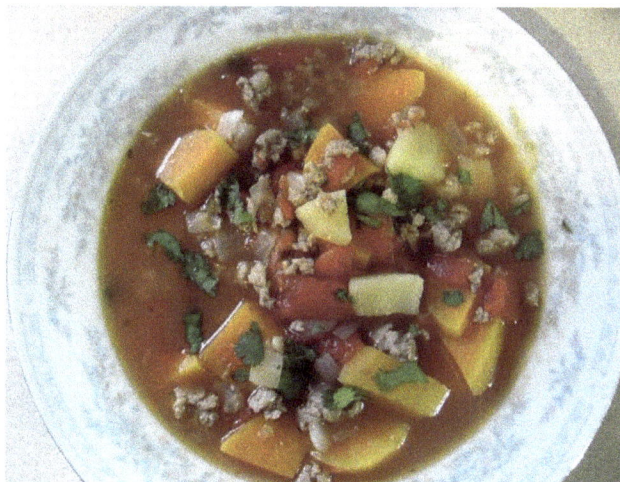

Preparation Time: 10 minutes

Cooking Time: 4 hours

Servings: 6

Ingredients:

- 1 1/2 lb. of chicken thighs, skinless and boneless

- 14 oz. of chicken stock

- 14 oz. of salsa

- 8 oz. of Monterey Jack cheese, shredded

Directions:

1. Place chicken into a Crock Pot.
2. Pour the remaining ingredients over the chicken.
3. Cover and cook on high for 4 hours.
4. Remove chicken from Crock Pot and shred using a fork.
5. Return shredded chicken to the Crock Pot and stir well.
6. Serve and enjoy.

Nutrition:

- Calories: 371
- Fat: 15 g
- Carbohydrates: 7 g
- Sugar: 2 g
- Protein: 41 g
- Cholesterol: 135 mg

Beef Stew

Preparation Time: 10 minutes

Cooking Time: 5 hours 5 minutes

Servings: 8

Ingredients:

- 3 lb. of beef stew meat; trimmed
- 1/2 cup of red curry paste
- 1/3 cup of tomato paste
- 13 oz. can of coconut milk
- 2 tsps. of ginger; minced
- 2 garlic cloves; minced
- 1 medium onion; sliced
- 2 tbsps. of olive oil
- 2 cups of carrots; julienned
- 2 cups of broccoli florets
- 2 tsps. of fresh lime juice
- 2 tbsps. of fish sauce
- 2 tsps. of sea salt

Directions:

1. Heat 1 tablespoon of oil in a pan over medium heat.
2. Brown the meat on all sides in the pan.
3. Add brown meat to a Crock Pot.
4. Add the remaining oil to the same pan and sauté the ginger, garlic, and onion over medium-high heat for 5 minutes.
5. Add coconut milk and stir well.
6. Transfer pan mixture to the Crock Pot.
7. Add the remaining ingredients apart from carrots and broccoli.
8. Cover and cook on high for 5 hours.
9. Add carrots and broccoli in the last 30 minutes of cooking.
10. Serve and enjoy.

Nutrition:

- Calories: 537
- Fat: 26 g
- Carbohydrates: 13 g
- Sugar: 16 g
- Protein: 54 g
- Cholesterol: 152 mg

Creamy Broccoli Cauliflower Soup

Preparation Time: 10 minutes

Cooking Time: 6 hours

Servings: 6

Ingredients:

- 2 cups of cauliflower florets; chopped

- 3 cups of broccoli florets; chopped

- 3 1/2 cups of chicken stock

- 1 large carrot; diced

- 1/2 cup of shallots; diced

- 2 garlic cloves; minced

- 1 cup of plain yogurt

- 6 oz. of cheddar cheese; shredded

- 1 cup of coconut milk

- Pepper

- Salt

Directions:

1. Add all ingredients except milk, cheese, and yogurt to a Crock Pot and stir well.
2. Cover and cook on low for 6 hours.
3. Purée the soup using an immersion blender until smooth.
4. Add cheese, milk, and yogurt and blend until smooth and creamy.
5. Season with pepper and salt.
6. Serve and enjoy.

Nutrition:

- Calories: 281
- Fat: 20 g
- Carbohydrates: 14 g
- Sugar: 9 g
- Protein: 11 g
- Cholesterol: 32 mg

Squash Soup

Preparation Time: 10 minutes

Cooking Time: 8 hours

Servings: 6

Ingredients:

- 2 lb. of butternut squash; peeled, chopped into chunks
- 1 tsp. of ginger, minced
- 1/4 tsp. of cinnamon
- 1 tbsp. of curry powder
- 2 bay leaves
- 1 tsp. of black pepper
- 1/2 cup of heavy cream
- 2 cups of chicken stock
- 1 tbsp. of garlic; minced
- 2 carrots; cut into chunks
- 2 apples; peeled, cored, and diced
- 1 large onion; diced
- 1 tsp. of salt

Directions:

1. Spray a Crock Pot inside with cooking spray.
2. Add all the ingredients except the cream to the Crock Pot and stir well.
3. Cover and cook on low for 8 hours.
4. Purée the soup using an immersion blender until smooth and creamy.
5. Stir in cream and season soup with pepper and salt.
6. Serve and enjoy.

Nutrition:

- Calories: 170
- Fat: 4 g
- Carbohydrates: 34 g
- Sugar: 14g
- Protein: 9 g
- Cholesterol: 14 mg

Butternut Squash Rice

Preparation Time: 10 minutes

Cooking Time: 20 minutes

Servings: 4

Ingredients:

- 1-pound of butternut squash
- 1 tablespoon of ghee
- 1 onion: diced
- 1 teaspoon of salt
- 1 oz. of fresh parsley; chopped
- 1 tablespoon of olive oil

Directions:

1. Chop the butternut squash into the rice pieces.
2. Put the ghee in the air fryer basket and add diced onion.
3. Sprinkle the onion with the salt and olive oil.
4. Cook it at $400°$ F for 2 minutes.
5. Then stir the onion and add the butternut squash rice.
6. Stir it and cook the meal for 18 minutes at $380°$ F.
7. Stir the squash every 4 minutes.

8. When the meal is cooked, sprinkle it with the chopped parsley and stir.

9. Serve it immediately!

Nutrition:

- Calories: 123
- Fat: 6.9 g
- Fiber: 3.1 g
- Carbs: 16.3 g
- Protein: 1.7 g

Roasted Apple with Bacon

Preparation Time: 20 minutes

Cooking Time: 10 minutes

Servings: 8

Ingredients:

- 6 apples

- 7 oz. of bacon; chopped

- ½ teaspoon of salt

- ½ teaspoon of paprika

- ½ teaspoon of ground black pepper

- 1 tablespoon of avocado oil

Directions:

1. Punch medium holes in the apples.
2. Mix together the chopped bacon, salt, paprika, ground black pepper, and avocado oil.
3. Stir the mixture.
4. Fill the apple holes with the bacon mixture.
5. Put the apples in the air fryer basket.
6. Cook the apples for 10 minutes at 380º F.

7. When the time has passed and the apples are cooked, chill them for 6 minutes and serve!

Nutrition:

- Calories: 224
- Fat: 10.9 g
- Fiber: 4.2 g
- Carbs: 23.7 g
- Protein: 9.7 g

Fennel Slices

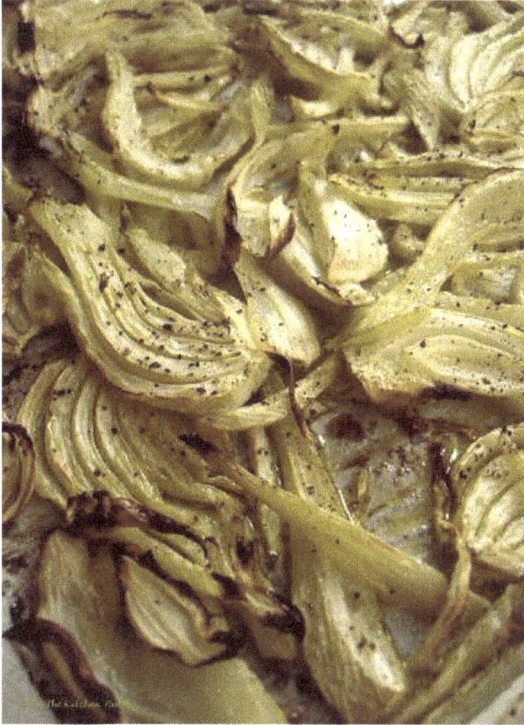

Preparation Time: 10 minutes

Cooking Time: 10 minutes

Servings: 2

Ingredients:

- 12 oz. of fennel bulb

- 1 teaspoon of paprika

- ½ teaspoon of chili flakes

- 1 tablespoon of olive oil

- 1 teaspoon of cilantro; dried

Directions:

1. Slice the fennel bulb and sprinkle it with the paprika, chili flakes, and dried cilantro on all sides.
2. Then sprinkle the fennel with the vegetable oil and transfer the vegetables to the air fryer basket.
3. Cook the fennel slices for 10 minutes at 380° F. Flip the fennel slices onto another side after 5 minutes of cooking.
4. Enjoy the cooked side dish!

Nutrition:

- Calories: 116
- Fat: 7.5 g
- Fiber: 5.7 g
- Carbs: 13 g
- Protein: 2.3 g

Eggplant Satay

Preparation Time: 15 minutes

Cooking Time: 18 minutes

Servings: 3

Ingredients:

- 3 eggplants
- 1 tablespoon of vinegar
- 1 tablespoon of olive oil
- 1 teaspoon of sesame seeds
- 1 teaspoon of dried dill
- ½ teaspoon of dried parsley
- ½ teaspoon of ground nutmeg

Directions:

1. Cut the eggplants into the cubes.
2. Then skew the eggplant onto the skewers.
3. Sprinkle the eggplants with the olive oil, vinegar, sesame seeds, dried dill, dried parsley, and ground nutmeg.

4. Place the eggplant satay in the air fryer basket and cook it for 18 minutes at 375° F.

5. When the eggplants are soft, the meal is cooked.

6. Let it chill a little and serve!

Nutrition:

- Calories: 187
- Fat: 6.3 g
- Fiber: 19.6 g
- Carbs: 32.9 g
- Protein: 5.7 g

Popcorn Mushrooms

Preparation Time: 10 minutes

Cooking Time: 10 minutes

Servings: 4

Ingredients:

- 16 oz. of mushrooms
- 2 tablespoons of almond flour
- 2 tablespoons of water
- ½ teaspoon of minced garlic
- 1 tablespoon of olive oil
- ¼ teaspoon of chili flakes

Directions:

1. Mix together the almond flour, water, minced garlic, and chili flakes in a bowl.
2. Stir the mixture.
3. Coat the mushrooms with the almond flour mixture.
4. Spray the olive oil inside the air fryer basket.
5. Put the mushrooms and cook them for 10 minutes at 365° F.

6. Stir the mushrooms every 2 minutes.

7. Serve the cooked popcorn mushrooms only hot!

Nutrition:

- Calories: 135
- Fat: 10.8 g
- Fiber: 2.6 g
- Carbs: 6.9 g
- Protein: 6.6 g

Thyme Mushrooms and Carrot Bowl

Preparation Time: 10 minutes

Cooking Time: 20 minutes

Servings: 4

Ingredients:

- 1 cup of baby carrot

- 8 oz. of mushrooms; sliced

- 1 teaspoon of thyme

- 1 teaspoon of salt

- 1 cup of chicken stock

- 1 teaspoon of chili flakes

- 1 teaspoon of coconut oil

Directions:

1. Place the baby carrot in the air fryer basket.
2. Add thyme, salt, and chili flakes.
3. Cook the baby carrot for 10 minutes at 380º F.
4. Then add the sliced mushrooms and coconut oil.

5. Stir it well and cook the vegetables for 10 minutes more at 370° F.
6. Stir the vegetables after 5 minutes of cooking.
7. Chill the cooked entremots and enjoy!

Nutrition:

- Calories: 25 g
- Fat: 1.5 g
- Fiber: 0.7 g
- Carbs: 2.2 g
- Protein: 2 g

Cinnamon Baby Carrot

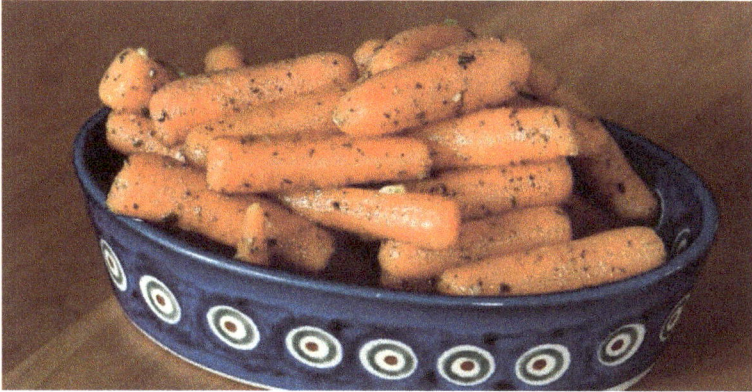

Preparation Time: 8 minutes

Cooking Time: 15 minutes

Servings: 4

Ingredients:

- 1-pound of baby carrot
- 1 tablespoon of ground cinnamon
- 1 teaspoon of ground ginger
- ¼ cup of almond milk
- 1 tablespoon of olive oil

Directions:

1. Wash the baby carrot carefully and sprinkle with the bottom cinnamon, ground ginger, and vegetable oil.
2. Stir the vegetables and transfer them to the air fryer basket.
3. Cook the baby carrot for 10 minutes at 380° F.
4. Then stir the baby carrots and add almond milk.
5. Stir the vegetables again and cook for 5 minutes more at the same temperature.
6. Let the cooked carrot chill a little and serve it!

Nutrition:

- Calories: 110 g
- Fat: 7.3 g
- Fiber: 4.6 g
- Carbs: 11.9 g
- Protein: 1.2 g

Chinese Eggplant with Chili and Garlic

Preparation Time: 10 minutes

Cooking Time: 24 minutes

Servings: 4

Ingredients:

- 2 eggplants
- 1 chili pepper; chopped
- 1 garlic clove; chopped
- ¼ teaspoon of ground coriander
- 1 tablespoon of olive oil
- ¼ teaspoon of salt
- 1 tablespoon of vinegar
- 3 teaspoon of water
- ¼ teaspoon of chili flakes

Directions:

1. Peel the eggplants and chop them.
2. Put the chopped eggplants in the air fryer basket.

3. Add chopped garlic, chili pepper, ground coriander, salt, and water.

4. Stir the vegetables and cook for twenty-four minutes at 365 º F.

5. When the eggplants are soft, transfer them to the bowl and sprinkle with the chili flakes and vinegar.

6. Stir well and serve immediately!

Nutrition:

- Calories: 101
- Fat: 4 g
- Fiber: 9.7 g
- Carbs: 16.5 g
- Protein: 2.8 g

Stuffed Eggplants with Cherry Tomatoes

Preparation Time: 15 minutes

Cooking Time: 25 minutes

Servings: 2

Ingredients:

- 1 eggplant

- 5 oz. of cherry tomatoes

- 1 shallot; chopped

- ½ teaspoon of salt

- ¾ teaspoon of nutmeg

- ¾ teaspoon of chili pepper

- 1 tablespoon of olive oil

Directions:

1. Cut the eggplant into the halves.
2. Remove the meat from the eggplants.
3. Chop the cherry tomatoes and mix them alongside the salt, shallot, nutmeg, chili pepper, and olive oil.
4. Stir the mixture.

5. Fill the eggplants with the vegetables.
6. Put the stuffed vegetables in the air fryer basket and cook for 25 minutes at 370º F.
7. Then chill the cooked eggplants a little.
8. Serve!

Nutrition:

- Calories: 136 g
- Fat: 7.9 g
- Fiber: 9.2 g
- Carbs: 16.9 g
- Protein: 3 g

Sesame Mushroom Slices

Preparation Time: 10 minutes

Cooking Time: 6 minutes

Servings: 3

Ingredients:

- 1 tablespoon of sesame seeds
- 1 tablespoon of avocado oil
- 14 oz. of mushrooms, sliced
- 1 teaspoon of chili flakes
- ¼ teaspoon of ground paprika

Directions:

1. Put the sliced mushrooms in the air fryer basket.
2. Add chili flakes and ground paprika.
3. Then add avocado oil and stir the mushrooms.
4. Cook the mushrooms for 4 minutes at 400° F. Stir the mushrooms after 2 minutes of cooking.
5. Sprinkle the mushrooms with the sesame seeds and stir well.

6. Cook the mushrooms for 2 more minutes at the same temperature.

7. Serve the mushrooms immediately!

Nutrition:

- Calories: 52 g
- Fat: 2.5 g
- Fiber: 2 g
- Carbs: 5.4 g
- Protein: 4.8 g

Leek Saute

Preparation Time: 10 minutes

Cooking Time: 15 minutes

Servings: 2

Ingredients:

- 10 oz. of leek, chopped

- 8 oz. of mushrooms; chopped

- 1 shallot; chopped

- 2 teaspoons of olive oil

- ¼ teaspoon of salt

- ½ teaspoon of chili flakes

1. **Directions:**
2. Put the chopped mushrooms in the air fryer basket.
3. Add olive oil and salt.
4. Then sprinkle the mushrooms with the chili flakes and stir well.
5. Cook the mushrooms for 5 minutes at 365° F.
6. Stir the mushrooms and add chopped shallot and leek.
7. Stir the vegetables.

8. Continue to cook the vegetables for 10 more minutes at 360º F.

9. Stir the vegetable time to time.

10. When all the ingredients are soft, the meal is cooked.

Nutrition:

- Calories: 151
- Fat: 5.4 g
- Fiber: 3.7 g
- Carb: 23.9 g
- Protein: 5.7 g

Sweet Potato Hasselback

Preparation Time: 15 minutes

Cooking Time: 35 minutes

Servings: 4

Ingredients:

- 4 sweet potatoes

- 4 garlic cloves; peeled

- ½ teaspoon of thyme

- 1 tablespoon of olive oil

- 1 teaspoon of dried basil

- ½ teaspoon of dried oregano

- 1 teaspoon of chili flakes

- 3 tablespoons of water

Directions:

1. Peel the sweet potatoes and cut them into the form of the Hasselback.

2. Put the sweet potatoes in the air fryer basket and cook them at 360° F for 20 minutes.

3. Meanwhile, mix together the thyme, olive oil, dried basil, dried oregano, chili flakes, and water.

4. Chop the garlic and add it to the mixture too.

5. Stir the spices.

6. Generously brush the Hasselback sweet potatoes with the spice mixture.

7. Cook the meal for 15 more minutes.

8. When the meal is cooked, let it chill a little.

9. Enjoy!

Nutrition:

- Calories: 36
- Fat: 3.6 g
- Fiber: 0.2 g
- Carbs: 1.3 g
- Protein: 0.2 g

Eggplant Lasagna

Preparation Time: 20 minutes

Cooking Time: 30 minutes

Servings: 3

Ingredients:

- 1 eggplant
- 2 tomatoes
- 1 tablespoon of olive oil
- 1 onion; diced
- 1 garlic clove; chopped
- 1 teaspoon of dried basil
- 1 teaspoon of ground black pepper
- ½ teaspoon of turmeric
- 1 teaspoon of cumin
- ½ cup of chicken stock
- 1 tablespoon of fresh dill; chopped
- 4 oz. of mushrooms; chopped

Directions:

1. Slice the eggplants.
2. Slice the tomatoes.
3. Mix together the diced onion, olive oil, chopped garlic, dried basil, ground black pepper, turmeric, cumin, and fresh dill in a bowl.
4. Stir the mixture.
5. Then make the layer of the sliced eggplants in the air fryer basket.
6. Sprinkle it with the spice mixture.
7. Put the tomatoes over the eggplants and add mushrooms.
8. Sprinkle the vegetables with the spice mixture and repeat all the steps till you are through with all the ingredients.
9. Add chicken broth and cook lasagna for 30 minutes at 365° F.
10. Let the cooked lasagna chill little and serve it!

Nutrition:

- Calories: 127 g
- Fat: 5.6 g
- Fiber: 8 g
- Carbs: 18.9 g
- Protein: 4.4 g

Ratatouille Kebabs

Preparation Time: 10 minutes

Cooking Time: 20 minutes

Servings: 4

Ingredients:

- 1 eggplant
- 1 sweet pepper
- 1 zucchini
- 1 onion; peeled
- 1 tomato
- 1 tablespoon of olive oil
- ½ teaspoon of chili flakes
- ½ teaspoon of ground coriander
- ½ teaspoon of salt

Directions:

1. Slice the eggplant, zucchini, and onion.
2. Cut the sweet pepper and tomato into the squares.
3. Skew the vegetables on the skewers.

4. Then sprinkle the vegetables with the olive oil, chili flakes, ground coriander, and salt.
5. Put the kebabs in the air fryer basket and cook for 20 minutes at 360° F.
6. Then gently transfer the cooked kebabs to the serving plate.
7. Enjoy!

Nutrition:

- Calories: 90
- Fat: 3.9 g
- Fiber: 5.8 g
- Carbs: 13.8 g
- Protein: 2.5 g

Parsley Zucchini and Radishes

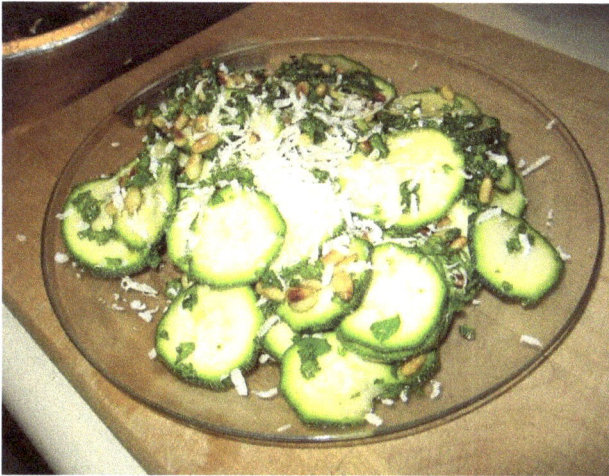

Preparation Time: 5 minutes

Cooking Time: 15 minutes

Servings: 4

Ingredients:

- 1 pound of zucchinis; cubed

- 1 cup of radishes; halved

- 1 tablespoon of olive oil

- 1 tablespoon of balsamic vinegar

- 2 tomatoes; cubed

- 3 tablespoons of parsley; chopped
- Salt and black pepper to the taste

Directions:

1. In a pan that matches your air fryer, mix the zucchinis with the radishes, oil, and the other ingredients, toss, introduce in the fryer and cook at 350º F for 15 minutes.
2. Divide between plates and serve with an entremots.

Nutrition:

- Calories 170
- Fat: 6 g
- Fiber: 2 g
- Carbs: 5 g
- Protein: 6 g

Cherry Tomatoes Sauté

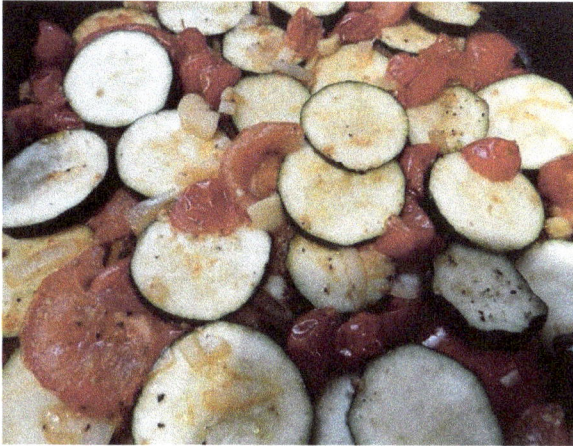

Preparation Time: 5 minutes

Cooking Time: 15 minutes

Servings: 4

Ingredients:

- 1 tablespoon of olive oil

- 1 pound of cherry tomatoes; halved

- Juice of 1 lime

- 2 tablespoons of parsley; chopped

- A pinch of salt and black pepper

Directions:

1. In a pan that fits the air fryer, mix the tomatoes with the oil and the other ingredients, toss, put the pan in the machine and cook at 360° F for 15 minutes.
2. Divide between plates and serve.

Nutrition:

- Calories: 141
- Fat: 6 g
- Fiber: 2 g
- Carbs: 4 g
- Protein: 7 g

Stuffed Tomatoes

Preparation Time: 20 minutes

Cooking Time: 15 minutes

Servings: 2

Ingredients:

- 7 oz. of mushrooms; chopped
- 1 teaspoon of minced garlic
- 1 tablespoon of fresh dill; chopped
- 1 onion; diced
- 2 tomatoes
- 1 tablespoon of olive oil
- ½ teaspoon of chili flakes

Directions:

1. Remove the meat from the tomatoes to form the tomato cups.
2. Mix together the chopped mushrooms, minced garlic, fresh dill, diced onion, olive oil, and chili flakes.
3. Stir the mixture well.

4. Fill the tomato cups with the mushroom mixture and put them in the air fryer.

5. Cook the entremots for 15 minutes at 360° F.

6. When the tomatoes are cooked, allow them to rest for 5 minutes and serve!

Nutrition:

- Calories: 132
- Fat: 7.7 g
- Fiber: 3.9 g
- Carbs: 14.5 g
- Protein: 5.2 g

Creamy Eggplant

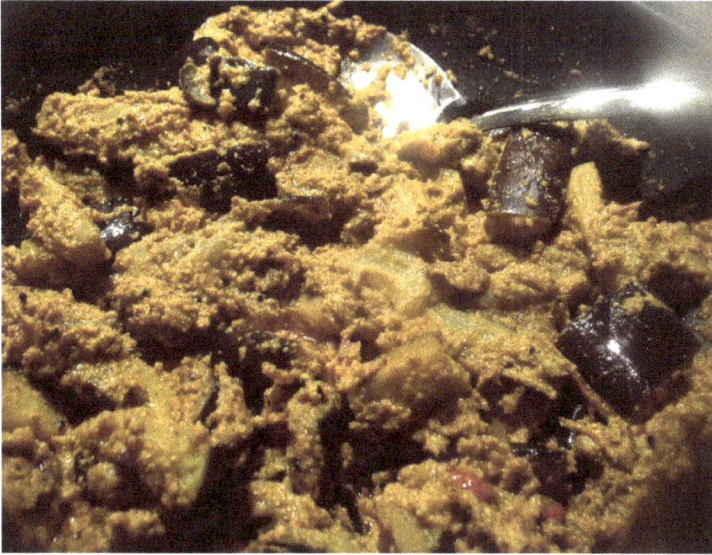

Preparation Time: 5 minutes

Cooking Time: 20 minutes

Servings: 4

Ingredients:

- 2 pounds of eggplants; roughly cubed

- 1 cup of heavy cream

- 2 tablespoons of butter; melted

- Salt and black pepper to the taste

- ½ teaspoon of chili powder

- ½ teaspoon of turmeric powder

Directions:

1. In a pan that fits the air fryer, mix the eggplants with the cream, butter, and the other ingredients, toss, put in the machine and cook at 370° F for 20 minutes.
2. Divide between plates and serve as a side dish.

Nutrition:

- Calories: 151
- Fat: 3 g
- Fiber: 2 g
- Carbs: 4 g
- Protein: 6 g

Parmesan Eggplants

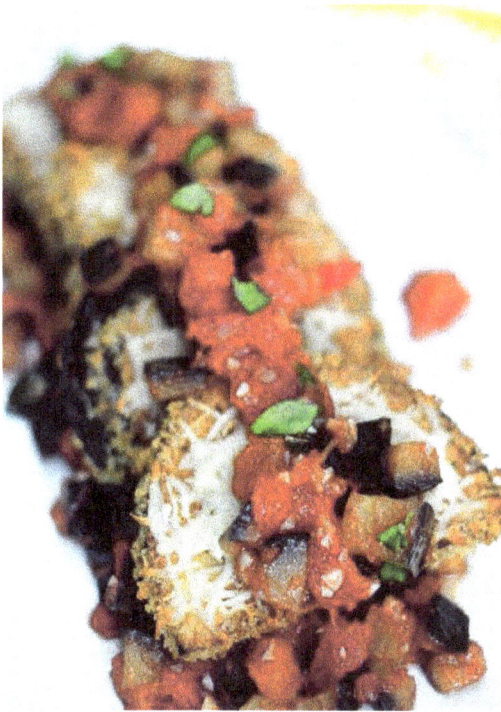

Preparation Time: 5 minutes

Cooking Time: 20 minutes

Servings: 4

Ingredients:

- 1 pound of eggplants; roughly cubed
- 1 tablespoon of olive oil

- 1 teaspoon of garlic powder

- 1 cup of parmesan; grated

- A pinch of salt and black pepper

- Cooking spray

Directions:

1. In the air fryer's pan, mix the eggplants with the oil and the other ingredients except the parmesan and toss.
2. Sprinkle the parmesan on top, put the pan in the machine and cook at 370° F for 20 minutes.
3. Divide between plates and serve as a side dish.

Nutrition:

- Calories: 183
- Fat: 6 g
- Fiber: 2 g
- Carbs: 3 g
- Protein: 8 g

Spaghetti Squash Casserole

Preparation Time: 10 minutes

Cooking Time: 20 minutes

Servings: 4

Ingredients:

- 12 oz. of spaghetti squash
- 1 teaspoon of ground cinnamon
- ½ teaspoon of salt
- 1 sweet potato; grated
- 1 tablespoon of almond flour
- 2 eggs
- 1 tablespoon of olive oil
- 1 onion; diced
- ¼ teaspoon of thyme

Directions:

1. Peel the spaghetti squash and chop it into ½ inch chunks.
2. Then place the squash in the air fryer basket.
3. Add salt and ground cinnamon.

4. Cook the sweet potatoes for 5 minutes at 380º F.

5. After this, make the layer of the grated potato over the sweet potato.

6. Beat the eggs in the bowl and whisk them.

7. Add almond flour and stir the mixture.

8. Then add olive oil, diced onion, and thyme.

9. Stir the mixture.

10. Pour it over the grated potato.

11. Cook the casserole for 15 minutes at 365º F.

12. When the time is over and casserole is cooked, let it chill little and serve!

Nutrition:

- Calories: 166
- Fat: 9.8 g
- Fiber: 2.6 g
- Carbs: 16.5 g
- Protein: 5.7 g

Kale Sauté

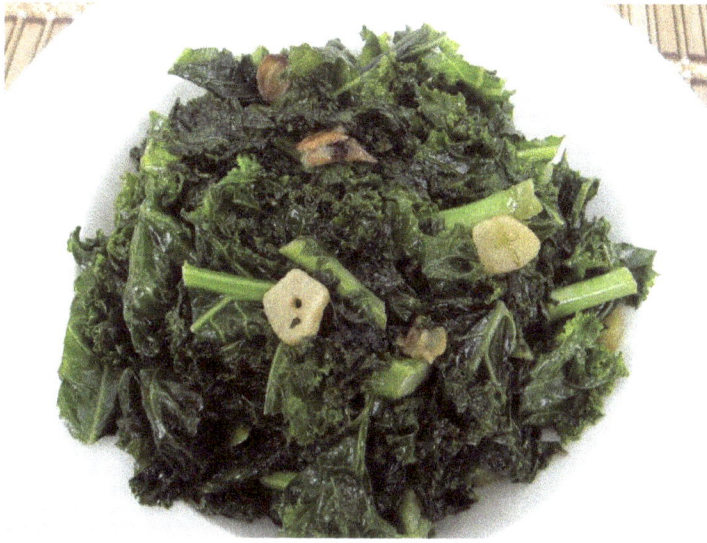

Preparation Time: 5 minutes

Cooking Time: 15 minutes

Servings: 4

Ingredients:

- 1 tablespoon of avocado oil

- 1 pound of baby kale

- ½ cup of heavy cream

- Salt and black pepper to the taste

97

- ¼ teaspoon of chili powder

- 1 tablespoon of dill; chopped

- ¼ cup of walnuts; chopped

Directions:

1. In a pan that fits the air fryer, mix the kale with the oil, cream, and the other ingredients, toss, put the pan in the machine and cook at 360º F for 15 minutes.
2. Divide between plates and serve as a side dish.

Nutrition:

- Calories: 160
- Fat: 7 g
- Fiber: 2 g
- Carbs: 4 g
- Protein: 5 g

Carrots Sauté

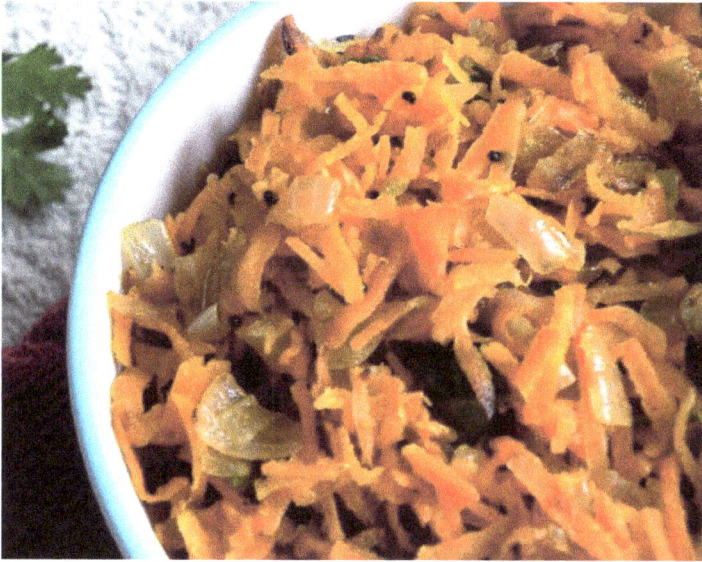

Preparation Time: 5 minutes

Cooking Time: 20 minutes

Servings: 4

Ingredients:

- 2 pounds of baby carrots; peeled

- 1 tablespoon of balsamic vinegar

- 2 tablespoons of olive oil

- Salt and black pepper to the taste

- 1 tablespoon of lemon juice

- 1/3 cup of almonds; chopped

- ½ cup of walnuts; chopped

Directions:

1. In a pan that fits the air fryer, mix the carrots with the vinegar, oil, and the other ingredients, toss, put the pan in the machine and cook at 380° F for 20 minutes.
2. Divide between plates and serve as a side dish.

Nutrition:

- Calories: 121
- Fat: 9 g
- Fiber: 2 g
- Carbs: 4 g
- Protein: 5 g

Eggplant Tongues

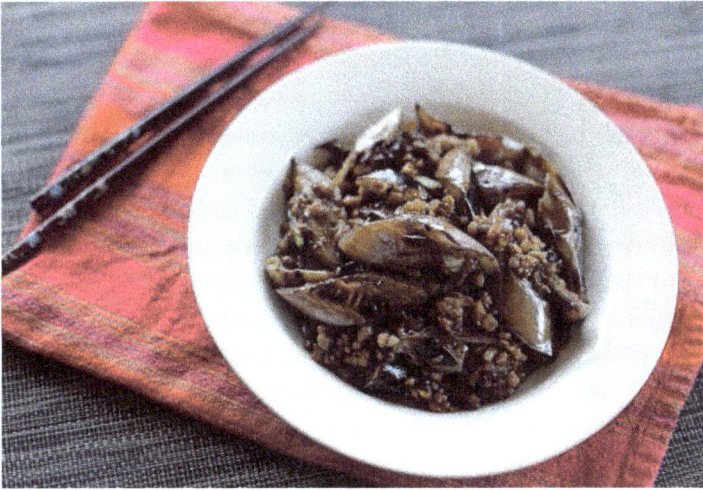

Preparation Time: 10 minutes

Cooking Time: 14 minutes

Servings: 2

Ingredients:

- 2 eggplants

- 1 teaspoon of minced garlic

- 1 teaspoon of olive oil

- ¼ teaspoon ground black pepper

Directions:

1. Wash the eggplants carefully and slice them.
2. Rub every eggplant slice with the minced garlic, olive oil, and ground black pepper.
3. Place the eggplants in the air fryer basket and cook for 7 minutes from all sides at 375º F.
4. When the eggplant tongues are cooked, serve them immediately!

Nutrition:

- Calories: 160
- Fat: 3.3 g
- Fiber: 19.4 g
- Carbs: 32.9 g

- Protein: 5.5 g

Eggplant and Carrots Mix

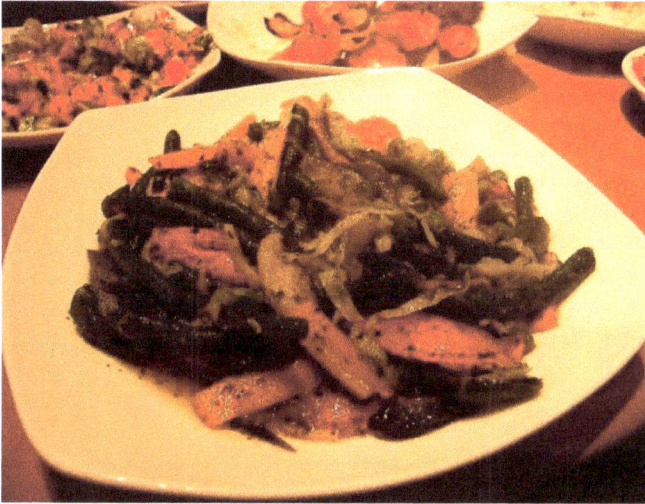

Preparation Time: 5 minutes

Cooking Time: 25 minutes

Servings: 4

Ingredients:

- 1 pound of eggplants; roughly cubed

- 1 pound of baby carrots

- 1 cup of heavy cream

- ½ teaspoon of chili powder

- 1 teaspoon of garlic powder

- 1 tablespoon of chives; chopped
- A pinch of salt and black pepper

Directions

1. In a pan that fits your air fryer, mix the eggplants with the carrots, cream and the other ingredients, toss, introduce in the air fryer and cook at 370 degrees F for 25 minutes.
2. Divide between plates and serve as a side dish.

Nutrition:

- Calories: 129
- Fat: 6 g
- Fiber: 2 g
- Carbs: 5 g
- Protein: 8 g

Bok Choy and Sprouts

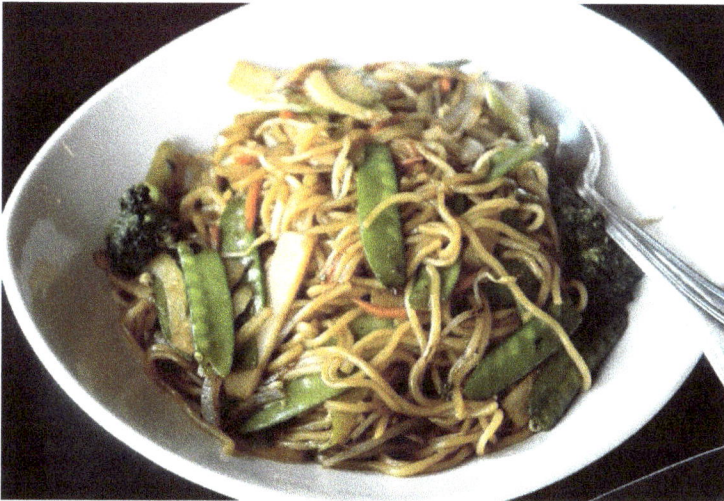

Preparation Time: 5 minutes

Cooking Time: 20 minutes

Servings: 4

Ingredients:

- 1 tablespoon of avocado oil
- 1 pound of Brussels sprouts; trimmed and halved
- 2 bok choy head; trimmed and cut into strips
- 1 tablespoon of balsamic vinegar
- A pinch of salt and black pepper

- 1 tablespoon of dill; chopped

Directions:

1. In a pan that fits your air fryer, mix the sprouts with the bok choy and the other ingredients, toss, put the pan in the air fryer and cook at 380° F for 20 minutes.
2. Divide between plates and serve as a side dish.

Nutrition:

- Calories: 141
- Fat: 3 g
- Fiber: 2 g
- Carbs: 4 g
- Protein: 3 g

Balsamic Radishes

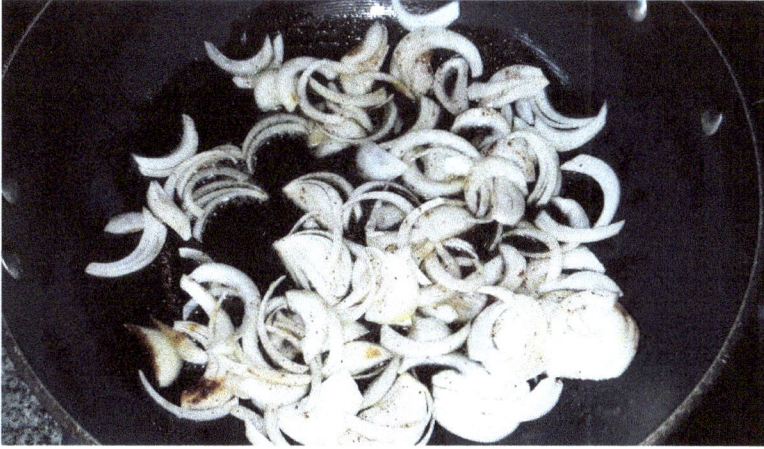

Preparation Time: 10 minutes

Cooking Time: 20 minutes

Servings: 4

Ingredients:

- 1 pound of radishes; halved
- 1 tablespoon of balsamic vinegar
- 1 teaspoon of chili powder
- 1 tablespoon of avocado oil
- Salt and black pepper to the taste

Directions:

1. In a pan that fits the air fryer, mix the radishes with the vinegar and the other ingredients, toss, put the pan in the air fryer and cook at 380° F for 20 minutes.
2. Divide between plates and serve as a side dish.

Nutrition:

- Calories: 151
- Fat: 2 g
- Fiber: 3 g
- Carbs: 5 g
- Protein: 5 g